Beyond Diet Recipes Book 3:

18 Easy Recipes For Fat Burn, Weight Loss and Optimal Health

By

Brittany Samons

Table of Contents

Beyond Diet Recipes Book 3:

18 Easy Recipes For Fat Burn, Weight Loss and Optimal Health

By Brittany Samons

First Published, 2014

Printed in the United States of America

Introduction

Keeping yourself in complete health is not an easy thing for sure, but it's not impossible. It just requires dedication and steadfastness. So, what to do to keep yourself healthy, fit and active? Well there are some of the things that must be done to ensure complete health:

1. Drinking water at least 8 – 12 glasses a day. It is good to drink more water early morning on empty stomach. The water keeps your body hydrated and help your metabolism to burn fat faster.

2. A regular routine of Walk: A routinely walk of an hour is also good enough to keep your metabolism active and helps your body to perform its functions efficiently.

3. A healthy eating habit: Taking the right nutrients and in balanced form is good enough to keep your body healthier and active. It will also help your body and brain to work in harmony. Make sure to cut off your calories intake to only required amount, as eating more than your daily requirement will only add up in the formation of fat in the body. Take more protein and less carbohydrates to build strong muscle and less fat layers.

4. Active Lifestyle: Make sure you are living an active life not static. The technological advancement has limited our various activities and bound us to sit in front of the computer for each and every work. Make sure to use the technology but in the right way. Limit your screen time and adopt some outdoor activity like sports, swimming, running etc.

5. Sleep: Sleep is another factor which is quite important to ensure a healthy life. Take 8 – 12 hours of sound sleep, as less sleep will deprived your body and mind activities by effecting the efficiency of your bodily functions. The sleep also play a vital role to burn fat so do not thing sleeping is the waste of time, but oversleeping is also bad. Make sure to take healthy sleeping hours.

Afore mentioned things if done in the routine greatly benefit you to keep yourself in complete health. Besides this, an important thing which must be taken seriously is adopting a healthy eating habit. Sometimes, it's quite hard to stay away from the delicious food and go for rough, boring and tasteless boiled food. But you do not need to worry any more, as these beyond diet recipes are not only providing you with healthy recipes, but also provide you with all the yummiest things you want to eat. So, try these calculated and healthy recipes and enjoy your life at its fullest.

1. Grilled Chicken Breast Recipe

Ingredients:

-1/4 cup of Olive Oil

- 1 lemon Juice

- 1 tablespoon of freshly ground pepper

- 4 boneless chicken breast (skinless)

- 1 teaspoon of salt

Instruction for Preparation:

First rinse the chicken properly under tap water. Take a bowl, put the chicken in it and ass lemon juice, pepper, salt and olive oil. Mix well with the chicken and place it in the refrigerator for an hour at least.

Now preheat the grill on medium flame. Place the chicken over the grill and cook it for 6 – 8 minutes then turn it and cook the other side until golden brown. Place the chicken in the plate and decorate with the salad and serve hot.

2. Slow Cooked Turkey Stew Recipe

Ingredients:

-1 medium sliced leek

- 2 teaspoon of fresh oregano

- 1 cup of peeled and cubed winter squash

- 1 stick of cinnamon

- Chicken stock or 2 cups of water

- 2 lb turkey pieces

- 2 teaspoon of fresh thyme leaves

- 1 medium chopped carrot

- 1 cup of cooked lentils

- 1 teaspoon of spike vegetable seasoning

- 16 oz. of diced tomatoes

Instructions for Preparation:

Take turkey and put in slow cooker placed on high by keeping the skin side down. Sauté it for 5 minutes until the fat het released. Now turn the side of turkey and add in it the fresh thyme, oregano, leek, spike and celery. Sauté it again until the leek get translucent. Now add the carrots, tomatoes, squash and cinnamon. Cover it and let it cook for 2 – 3 hours on low heat.

Once the chicken is done. Remove the cinnamon stick and add in it the cooked lentils. Stir all the ingredients well and serve hot in a bowl.

3. Stir Fry Turkey Recipe

Ingredients:

-1 large minced garlic clove

- 3 slice of fresh minced ginger root

- 1 medium cut in half round slices carrot

- 3 cups of chopped spinach or kale

- 1 medium chopped red onion

- 2 medium peeled and diced kohlrabi

- 2 cups of cooked turkey

- 2 teaspoon of dried thyme

- ¼ teaspoon of curry powder

- 8 0z. of freshly sliced mushrooms

- 1 peeled and sliced broccoli stem

- 1 cup of broccoli florets

-2 cups of sliced celery

- 1 tablespoon of coconut oil or butter

- 1 tablespoon of tamari

Instructions to Follow:

Take a heavy skillet and put it over a high flame. Add in it butter or coconut oil to heat. Now add in it the garlic and ginger. Sauté them by constant stirring for 45 seconds. Then add in it the broccoli stem, carrot, onions, kohlrabi and celery; fry them by stirring for 3 – 4 minutes at least. When the vegetables colors get brighten, add in it the mushrooms, broccoli florets and kale. Stir them and fry for 1 minute.

Now add in the thyme, cooked turkey and curry powder. Cover the pan and lower down the heat to medium. Let it cook for 2 minutes. Once all the vegetables get tender, turn off the heat and add in it tamari. Mix it well with other ingredients. Take a large plate and serve hot. Enjoy the full of nutrients, healthy diet instantly.

4. White Bean and Tomatoes Soap Recipe

Ingredients:

-8 cups of water

- 6 branches of fresh thyme or ½ tablespoon of dried thyme

- 3 tablespoon of olive oil

- 1 medium chopped onion

- ½ cup of washed, soaked dry white beans

- 1 pound of fresh tomatoes

- 3 bay leaves

- 1 teaspoon of salt, or to taste

- 4 peeled garlic cloves

- 10 sage leaves

Instructions for preparation:

Wash, drain and rinse the white beans. Put them in a bowl full of water and add in it the thyme leaves, 3 garlic cloves, 2 bay leaves, 5 sage leaves and 1 tablespoon of oil. Put the bowl over medium heat and let it boil. Now add in it the salt and lower down the heat and let the beans to cook or boil for an hour until they get tender. Now remove the garlic, bay, thyme and sage from the bowl. The water and beans must be kept aside.

Tale a pan and put it on the medium heat. Add in it the remaining oil along with the sage, bay and minced garlic clove. Sauté them for 1 minute, then add in it the onion and sauté again by constant stirring for 10 minutes or until the onion got translucent.

Now add in it the tomatoes, bean water and salt. Cook them for 20 minutes. Now add in it the already cooked beans and let it boil for 10 minutes.

Take a bowl and pour the hot white beans and tomatoes soup in it. Serve it hot. You can even store it in refrigerator. Let it cool down then pour it in the airtight jar and keep it in the refrigerator. The taste of soup will get improve over the couple of days.

5. Egg Salad Recipe

Ingredients:

-2 finely chopped green onions

- 1 ½ tablespoon of mustard

- Salt to taste

- 2 peeled hard boiled eggs

- 1 tablespoon of lemon juice

- Ground black pepper to taste

- 1 teaspoon of Worcestershire sauce

Directions to Follow:

Take a medium sized bow. Add in it the eggs and mashed it using the fork. Now add in it the green chopped onions and mix well. Then add into the bowl, salt, pepper, mustard, lemon juice and Worcestershire sauce. Mix all the ingredients together using a spoon. Cover the bowl and put it in the refrigerator overnight. Next day enjoy the healthiest breakfast.

6. Cooked or Boiled Beans Recipe

Ingredients:

-1 cup of dried bean (of any type but preferable red or black)
- Water as per requirement

Instructions for Preparation:

Take the dried beans and wash them with the water. Boil the water and put the beans in it. Soaked the beans in the boiling water for 1 – 2 hours. When they get doubled in size and wrinkle free, drain the water and rinse the beans again. Take a saucepan and add the bean in it. Put the water and salt in it. Cover the sauce pan and let it cook on medium flame until beans get tender. If you are using pressure cooker then cook for 10 – 15 minutes in the pressure cooker on medium flame.

Once the beans get tender and soft. Turn off the heat and use the bean in salads, soups and anything you want. Put the bean in a bowl and cover it with the plastic wrapper. Place the bowl in the refrigerator for 2 days and use as per requirement. Following this recipe you can cook the beans and can store them in the refrigerator to quickly make delicious salads and soups. Beans are full of protein and a quite healthy ingredient for the people looking for weight loss. So add the beans in your diet and live a healthy and fit life.

7. Salmon Ceviche Recipe

Ingredients:

-1 cup of fresh lime juice

- 2 teaspoon of salt

- 2 cups of chopped parsley

- 1 lb of Salmon

- 2 tablespoon of freshly chopped and seeded Serrano pepper

- ½ cup of diced red onion

- 1 cup of chopped tomatoes

Instructions for Preparation:

Tale salmon and chopped into ½ - ¼ inch pieces. Now mix with the salmon, onion, pepper, salt and lime juice. Set salmon aside to marinate for several hours or overnight.

Before serving add in it the chopped tomatoes and cilantro and mix well. Then serve in a bowl. Make sure to mix tomatoes and cilantro before 20 minutes of serving.

8. Low Fat Chicken Salad Recipe

Ingredients:

-1 teaspoon of finely chopped parsley

- 2 teaspoon of mustard

- 2 dashes of hot pepper sauce

- Ground black pepper to taste

- 4 oz. of chicken breast

- 1 tablespoon of chopped and sliced almonds

- 2 tablespoon of chicken stock

- salt to taste

- ¼ cup of chopped celery

Directions to Prepare:

Take a medium bowl and add in it the chicken breasts cut into cubical small pieces, chopped almonds, parsley and celery. Mix all the ingredients well. Tale another bowl and put in it the stock, pepper sauce and mustard. Whisk them well. Now combine the mixtures of the both bowls and stir them. Season them with the grounded black pepper and salt. Enjoy the healthy chicken salad.

9. Marinated Pork Chop Recipe

Ingredients:

-2 minced garlic cloves

- 1 cup of white wine

- Sea Salt to taste

- Finely ground black pepper to taste

- 3 teaspoon of paprika

- 6 pork chops

Instructions for Preparation:

Take an oven dish and layer it with the pork pieces. Take a bowl and add in it the paprika, garlic, salt and pepper. Mix all the contents well and spread it over the pork chops in the baking dish. Now pour the white wine over the pork chops. Now cover the baking dish and let it stay in refrigerator for at least 6 hours.

Now preheat the oven at 300F. Now take off the baking dish from the refrigerator and place it into the oven and bake it until the pork get tender and turn into golden brown color. Turn off the oven and take off the dish. Serve the hot pork chops in a plate with finely cut cucumber, tomatoes and some lettuce leaves.

10. Roasted Lamb Leg Recipe

Ingredients:

-1/4 cup of soy sauce

- 1 minced garlic clove

- 2 tablespoon of olive oil

- 1 6 – 8 lb. leg of lamb

- 1 tablespoon of freshly minced rosemary

- 1 peeled and minced fresh piece of ginger root (1 inch)

- ½ cup of mustard

Instruction for Preparation:

First of all preheat the oven at 350F. Now take a bowl and add in it the ginger, minced garlic, rosemary, mustard and soy sauce. Mix all these ingredients well. Add in it the oil and whisk to make a creamy mixture, now set aside the bowl.

Take the lamb leg and with the help of a knife mark in at 3 – 4 places. Now put a slice of garlic in each mark. Now brush the mixture prepared previously on the lamb leg. Keep it aside for an hour.

Now roast the lamb on the rack placed in the oven for 1 – ½ hour. When the lamb meat get tender and turn into golden brown color. Turn off the oven and take off the rack. Serve the hot lamb by seasoning it with the lemon juice and salad.

11. Peanut Butter Banana Oat Breakfast Cookies Recipe

Ingredients:

-2/3 cup of unsweetened apple sauce

- 1 teaspoon of vanilla extract

- ¼ cup of chopped nuts

- 2 mashed and creaming bananas

- ¼ cup of chocolate chips

- 1/3 cup of peanut butter

- 1 scoop of vanilla protein powder

- 1 ½ cups of oats

Instructions for Preparation:

First of all heat the oven at 350 F. Take a large bowl and mashed the banana in it until turn into the creamy paste. Now add in it the peanut butter and mix them well. Then add in it the vanilla extract, unsweetened apple sauce and vanilla protein powder. Stir them all together well until combined.

Now add in the chocolate chips, nuts and oatmeal and mix them all well. Now a dough will be formed. Let this dough stay for 10 minutes. Take the parchment cookie paper and using spoon put some dough on it, then shape it like cookies on parchment paper. Repeat the same until all the dough turn into the round cookies.

Take a baking dish and lined these cookies in it. Put the baking dish in to the oven and let it bake for 20 – 30 minutes or until they turn into the golden brown. Remove the baking dish from the oven and let the cookies to cool down for 5 minutes before placing on cookies rack for further cooling.

Once the cookies are cool completely, put them into an air tight jar and store them for use as per requirements.

12. Black Beans Veggies Burger Recipe

Ingredients:

-1/2 cup of finely chopped green pepper

- 1 large chopped celery stalk

- 1 teaspoon of cumin

- ¼ teaspoon of cayenne pepper

- 1/3 cup of hummus

- 2 slices of SWG fresh bread

- 2 cup of cooked black beans

- ½ cup of finely chopped red onion

- 1 – 2 minced garlic cloves

- 1 tablespoon of cooking oil

- salt to taste

- ½ cup of oats

- Ground black pepper to taste

Directions to Prepare:

Take the fresh SWG bread and crumbles it into the tiny pieces using the food processor. Take a bowl and add in it the cooked red beans which are turned into puree using the food processor. Also ass in it the red onion, salt, pepper, chopped celery, cayenne pepper, cumin, garlic, oats and chopped green peppers. Mix all the ingredients well.

Take the mixture and shape it like a big round cookie. Put the pan over a medium heat and add in it the cooking oil. Now cook the mixture cookie in the pan until turn into the golden brown or cook well. It may take 10 – 15 minutes.

Turn it and cook the other side too. Now take the bun pieces and sauté them into little oil in the pan. Place the mixture cookie between the two pieces of bun and also place the freshly cut tomatoes and you can also use mayonnaise or ketchup too. Enjoy the nutrients full hot black bean and veggie burger.

13. Tea Juice Recipe

Ingredients:

-3 quarts of boiling water

- Stevia powder to taste

- 5 – 6 bags of caffeine free herbal tea (fruit, mint, peach or chamomile tea)

Directions for Preparation:

Take a large pot or glass and place the tea bags in it Put the boiling water over the tea bags and add in it the stevia. Mix them well and adjust it taste until desired sweetness is attained. Now let the tea get cool. Remove the tea bags from the pot and pour it in the serving glasses. Place it in the refrigerator to cool down. Enjoy the healthy tea juice and live a fit life.

14. Lentil Rice Slow Cooker Soup Recipe

Ingredients:

-2 cups of uncooked brown rice long grain

- ½ cup of chopped celery stalk

- ½ chopped or diced onion

- 1 cup of vegetable broth

- ½ teaspoon of freshly ground black pepper, or to

taste

- 1 cup of freshly sliced mushrooms

- 2 cups of dry lentils

- 1 cup of chopped baby carrots

- 8 cups of water

- 1 teaspoon of garlic powder

- 1 tablespoon of Sea salt or to taste

Instructions for preparation:

Take a pressure cooker. Drain and rinse the lentils and
rice. Put them in the cooker. Add in it the 8 cups of the
water. Now add in it the chopped onions, celery,
carrots, garlic powder, salt, black pepper and vegetable
broth in it. Now place the pressure cooker on the low
heat and let it cook for 7 – 8 hours. Once the rice is
cooked and lentils get tender. Turn off the heat and

stir in it the freshly sliced mushrooms before an hour of serving.

Take a bowl and pour in it the hot lentil rice soup and enjoy in cold winter nights the protein full diet to keep you healthy and active.

15. Breakfast Burritos Recipe

Ingredients:

-1/2 cup of freshly chopped onions

- 1 – 2 tablespoon of freshly minced thyme or rosemary

- ½ cup of chopped pecans or walnuts

- SWG tortillas

- 1 – 2 tablespoon of butter

- 2 – 3 eggs

- 2 tablespoon of soy sauce

- 1 chopped small tomato

- 2 – 3 tablespoon of grated cheese

Directions to Prepare:

Take a pan and put it on the medium heat. Add in it the onion and butter. Sauté the onions until they get translucent or for 3 – 4 minutes. Take a bowl and scramble the eggs in it. Now pour the eggs into the sautéed onions. Let it cook or 2 minutes by constant stirring.

Now add in it the soy sauce, thyme and tomatoes. Stir them well and let it become warm. Then add in it the grated cheese and chopped walnuts. Stir them and remove the pan from the heat.

Take the SWG tortilla and put this mixture with the help of the spoon at the center of the tortilla. Fold the ends and make it look like a roll. Repeat the same procedure for all the SWG tortillas or till the mixture get ends. Here you go with the delicious and nutrients filled breakfast to kick start your day.

16. Turkey Chili Recipe

Ingredients:

-1 lb. of ground turkey

- 1 cup of chopped red bell pepper

- 2/3 cup of coarsely chopped celery

- 2 teaspoon of chili powder

- 1 teaspoon of ground cumin

- 14 ½ oz. chopped plum tomatoes

- 1 bay leaf

- 2 teaspoon of butter

- salt to taste

- 1 chopped medium onion

- 1 minced garlic clove

- 1 teaspoon of paprika

- ½ teaspoon ground cayenne pepper

- ½ of chicken stock

- Freshly ground black pepper to taste

Directions for Preparation:

Take a pan and put it over high heat, add in it the 1 teaspoon of the butter. Now add in it the turkey, salt and grounded black pepper. Cook them with constant stirring for 2 – 3 minutes or until the turkey turn into the golden brown color. Now remove the pan from the stove. Take off the turkey in a bowl and cover it to keep it warn. Set it aside.

Now again put the pan on the low heat and add in it the 1 teaspoon of butter. When the butter melt down, add in it the chopped onions, red pepper, garlic and celery. Let them cook until all the vegetables get tender or cook it for 3 – 5 minutes at least.

Now add in it the paprika, cumin, chili powder and cayenne. Stir them well and let it cook for a minute. Now increase the heat under the pan and add in it the bay leaf, chicken stock and tomatoes. Cook them while stirring until it starts to boil. Lower down the heat and let it cook for 15 minutes.

Once the tomatoes get cooked well, add in it the cooked turkey from the bowl. Stir it and let it cook for 5 minutes. Now remove the pan from the heat and take off the cooked turkey in a plate. Remove the bay leaf and serve the turkey chili hot.

17. Broiled Lemon Salmon Recipe

Ingredients:

-1 minced garlic clove

- 1 teaspoon of olive oil

- 4 – 6 ounces of salmon fillets

- 1 tablespoon of tamari

- ½ cup of fresh lemon juice

- 2 tablespoon of chopped chives

- 1 whole lemon cut it into slices

Instructions for Preparation:

Take a bowl and add in it the lemon juice, garlic, olive oil, tamari and chives. Whisk them all together. Now take the salmon fillets and pour over it this mixture. Let it marinate for 20 – 30 minutes.

Now put the salmon with the layer of lemon slices underneath to broil. Let it broil for 3- 4 minutes and turn its side to golden brown the other side as well. Check with the form whether the salmon get cooked deep or not. Take off the salmon in the serving plate. Place the slices of broiled lemon over the broiled salmon fillets. Serve it hot. You can also put the salad in the plate to make it more nutritional full meal. Cut some fresh tomatoes and cucumber into slices. First place the lettuce leave in the plate then place the slices of tomatoes and cucumber at one side of the plate. Put the salmon fillets over the remaining area on the leaves and season it with the lemon. Enjoy the mouthwatering broiled lemon salmon.

18. Herb and Garlic Marinated Chicken Breast Recipe

Ingredients:

-1 teaspoon of dried thyme

- 1 teaspoon of dried tarragon

- 1 teaspoon of ground black pepper

- ½ cup of olive oil

- 1 tablespoon of olive oil

- 5 minced garlic cloves

- 1 teaspoon of dried oregano

- 1 lemon (juice)

- 6 boneless chicken breast cut into the halves

- 1 teaspoon of salt

- 1 teaspoon of dried basil

Instructions to Prepare:

Take a bowl and add in it the dried herbs, salt, pepper, garlic, lemon juice and olive oil. Mix them all well. Now take the chicken breast and apply this mixture on the chicken breast. Place them into the refrigerator for at least 2 hours to marinate.

Now preheat the grill on high flame. Brush the grate with the olive oil. Place the chicken breast one get marinated well over the grate for 5 minutes per side or until turn golden brown.

Remove the breast from the grate and place it on the serving plate and enjoy hot the chicken breast with garlic and herbs.

Final Words

Although eating rightly can help you maintain your health and weight, but if you are facing weight challenges and looking to lose some, then it's better to adopt some healthy and productive activities like walking and exercise. This will ensure prevention of further fat deposit and will also shed the already present one. It needs patience to acquire the desire results and consistent efforts towards keeping your life in complete balance by eating healthy and adopting a healthy life style. Avoid the consumption of fast food and soft drinks, surely they taste good but they are fat welcoming food. Having a good control over yourself is also a good thing to learn, if you really want to live a healthy long life.

So, now cook the right meal for yourself and prepare your diet plan to live a healthy life which will not only provide with you healthy body but mind too. Most importantly, you will feel satisfy and confident while socializing without facing any fear about your body. Let's start to get a healthy slim body and try out some of these amazing beyond diet recipes to ensure complete healthy meals being part of your diet regime.

Thank You Page

I want to personally thank you for reading my book. I hope you found information in this book useful and I would be very grateful if you could leave your honest review about this book. I certainly want to thank you in advance for doing this.

Lightning Source UK Ltd.
Milton Keynes UK
UKOW06f1848030815

256316UK00014B/615/P

9 781680 329063